THE COMPLETE GUIDE TO USING CIPROFLOXACIN

The Step by Step Guide Used to Treat and Prevent Bacterial Infections Such as Pneumonia,Gonorrhea,Typhoid Fever,Infectious Diarrhea,Bronchitis,Sinus Infections,Urinary Tract Infections and Plague

ISBN 978-1-0879-5158-4

Pavon Brown

TABLE OF CONTENT

CHAPTER 1

INTRODUCTION

When used to treat or prevent certain
infections caused by bacteria, such as
pneumonia, gonorrhea (a sexually
transmitted disease), typhoid fever (a
serious infection common in developing
countries), infectious diarrhea
(infections that cause severe diarrhea),
and infections of the skin, bone, joint,
abdomen (stomach area), and prostate,
ciprofloxacin is known as a beta-lactam
antibiotic (male reproductive gland), It
is also used to treat or prevent plague
(a deadly infection that might be
disseminated on purpose as part of a
bioterrorist assault) and anthrax
inhalation (a kind of anthrax that is
transferred via the air) (a serious

infection that may be spread by anthrax germs in the air on purpose as part of a bioterror attack). It may also be used to treat bronchitis, sinus infections, and urinary tract infections, although it should not be used to treat bronchitis and sinus infections, as well as some forms of urinary tract infections, if there are better treatment choices available. Some types of urinary tract infections should only be treated with ciprofloxacin extended-release (long-acting) tablets if there are no other treatment options available. Ciprofloxacin extended-release (long-acting) tablets are used to treat kidney and urinary tract infections; however, they should only be used when there are no other treatment options available. Ciprofloxacin is an antibiotic that belongs to a family of medicines known as fluoroquinolones.

Colds, flu, and other viral diseases will not be treated with antibiotics such as ciprofloxacin, for example. Taking antibiotics when they are not necessary raises your chances of having an infection that is resistant to antibiotic treatment later on in life.

CHAPTER 2

Concerning the antibiotic ciprofloxacin

Hexafluoroquinolone is an antibiotic that belongs to the fluoroquinolone class of medicines.

It is used to treat dangerous infections or illnesses that have failed to respond to previous antibacterial treatments.

It is employed in the treatment of bacterial illnesses such as:

Infections of the lungs (including pneumonia)

Infections of the skin and bones

Infections that are transferred by sexual contact (STIs)

Conjunctivitis is an infection of the eyes.

Ear infections are a common problem.

It can be used to assist prevent people from contracting meningitis if they have been in close proximity to someone who has contracted the sickness.

Ciprofloxacin is only available through a physician's referral.

It is available in a variety of forms, including pills, a liquid to drink, eardrops, eyedrops, and an eye ointment. It can also be administered as an injection, however this is normally done in a hospital setting.

Because of the possibility of major side effects, ciprofloxacin pills and liquid are not used as frequently as certain other forms of antibiotics.

The most important information

Nitrates and diarrhea are the most prevalent adverse effects of ciprofloxacin pills and liquid, with nausea and vomiting being the most common.

If you're taking the pills or liquid with dairy items like milk, cheese, or yoghurt, avoid eating them together.

There has been a rare report of the pills and liquid causing weak muscles, soreness or tingling in your legs and arms, painful or swollen joints and tendons, and an abnormally rapid or irregular heartbeat in some people. If any of these things happen to you, get medical attention right once.

Ciprofloxacin is also known by the brand names Ciproxin (tablets and liquid), Ciloxan (eyedrops and eye ointment), and Cetraxal (eye drops and eye ointment). Ciprofloxacin is used to treat infections caused by bacteria (eardrops).

Ciprofloxacin eardrops are also available in combinations with other medications, such as dexamethasone (marketed under the brand name Cetraxal Plus) and fluocinolone (known as Cilodex).

3. Who should not take ciprofloxacin and who should

Ciprofloxacin can be taken by the majority of adults and children starting at the age of one year and older.

Some people should avoid using Ciprofloxacin because of its side effects.

Tell your doctor if you have any of the following conditions to ensure that ciprofloxacin is safe for you:

If you have ever had an allergic reaction to ciprofloxacin or any other medication, or if you have ever experienced a major adverse effect from ciprofloxacin or another antibiotic, you should not use it (particularly a fluroquinolone) If you have ever experienced diarrhea after taking antibiotics, or if you or a member of your family has an abdominal aortic aneurysm or any other issue with the aorta, you should consult your doctor (the large blood vessel running from the heart to the abdomen)

Your heart is racing, thumping, or irregularly beating.

Have a heart infection, congenital heart disease, or heart valve disease; have uncontrolled high blood pressure; or have a combination of the above.

If you have rheumatoid arthritis, Behcet's illness, or a connective tissue problem such as Marfan syndrome, you should consult your doctor.

In the event that you have tendon difficulties, you may also have epilepsy or another medical condition that puts you at risk of having seizures.

You are experiencing difficulties with your kidneys.

If you have diabetes, you should avoid using ciprofloxacin since it may cause your blood sugar levels to rise.

CHAPTER 3

What to take and when to take it

The way you take your medicine is determined by the type of ciprofloxacin you're taking and the purpose for which you're taking it.

Make an effort to distribute the dosages equally throughout the day. Unless your doctor instructs you otherwise, continue taking or using this medication until the course is completed.

How should the pills and fluids be consumed?

Ciprofloxacin is available in three dosage strengths: 250mg, 500mg, and 750mg. It is also available as a liquid, with a 5ml spoonful containing 250mg (250mg/5ml) of the medication.

Ciprofloxacin is typically taken twice a day in doses ranging from 250mg to 750mg. Some illnesses may only need the administration of a single dosage.

****

Children and people with renal difficulties are often given lesser doses than the general population.

Take the pills whole, with plenty of water, and swallow them. Do not consume them whole.

Ciprofloxacin liquid is delivered in the form of granules that must be dissolved in the particular liquid given. Follow the directions on the label of the medication you're taking.

Shake the container of ciprofloxacin liquid for 15 seconds before using it to ensure that all of the granules have been dissolved.

The liquid is packaged with a plastic syringe or spoon to assist you in obtaining the proper dosage. If you do not have one, you can obtain one from your pharmacist. A kitchen teaspoon should not be used since it will not deliver the correct dosage.

Ciprofloxacin pills and liquid can be taken with or without food, depending on your preference. However, dairy products such as milk, cheese, and yoghurt should be avoided since they might interfere with the effectiveness of your medication.

Instructions on how to use the eyedrops

Four times a day, you'll normally apply 1 or 2 drops into the eye that's been impacted.

If you have a serious illness, your doctor may advise you to use the drops as frequently as every 15 minutes during the first 6 hours after the infection occurs. You will then be able to minimize the frequency with which you utilize it.

Pulling down your lower eyelid with a clean finger and tilting your head back will help you relax.

Holding the bottle above your eye, allow a single drop to fall into the gap between your lower lid and your eye is a good starting point.

Remove any excess liquid by wiping it away with a clean tissue.

If you have been instructed to put in a second drop, do so.

The dropper should not be used to contact your eye or eyelid since it may cause infection to spread.

The proper way to apply eye ointment

Apply a little more than 1 cm of ointment to the afflicted eye twice or three times a day, or as directed by your doctor. If the infection is severe, your doctor may advise you to use it as frequently as every hour and throughout the night, even if the illness is minor.

Pulling down your lower eyelid with a clean finger and tilting your head back will help you relax.

Gently squeeze the ointment into the gap between your lower lid and your eye, while maintaining contact with the tip of the tube close to your eye.

You should avoid touching your eye or your eyelid with the nozzle since this might cause infection to spread.

What to do with the eardrops

Fill the afflicted ear with up to 5 drops of the prescribed medication twice a day, or as directed by your doctor.

Holding the container in your hands for a few minutes will help to warm up the droplets.

Raise your head and bring the container up to your afflicted ear, with the open end of the container close to the opening of your ear hole.

Fill your ear with the drops by squeezing them.

If at all possible, try to get some rest for at least 5 minutes thereafter.

If you are only treating one ear, tilt your head to one side so that the ear that is being treated is towards the ceiling.

What happens if I don't remember to take it?

It's best to take a missed dosage as soon as you recall it rather than waiting until your next dose is scheduled. In this situation, simply skip the missing dose and continue with your regular schedule for the following dose.

Make certain that you complete the entire course of antibiotics.

If you tend to forget to take your medication on a regular basis, setting an alarm to remind you may be beneficial. You might also consult with your pharmacist for suggestions on alternative methods of keeping track of your medications.

What happens if I ingest or use too much of something?

It is perfectly OK to use too much eye ointment, eye or eardrops if you are applying them to the eyes or ears. In most cases, this will not result in any issues.

Ciprofloxacin pills or liquid are both options.

If you consume more of the pills or liquid than is recommended, you may have negative effects. Some of these are nausea or vomiting, diarrhoea, and a pounding or erratic heartbeat, among other things. If you suffer from epilepsy, you may experience seizures or fits.

CHAPTER 4

Symptoms and side consequences

It is possible to get adverse effects with ciprofloxacin just like any other medication, however not everyone does.

Consequences that are common

More than 1 in every 100 persons will experience one or more of the common adverse effects of ciprofloxacin. Inform your doctor if any of the following adverse effects persist or do not go away:

feelings of nausea or vomiting after taking the tablets or liquid vomiting and diarrhea after taking the tablets or liquid red or uncomfortable eyes with a stinging, burning, or gritty feeling after using the eyedrops or ointment

After using the eyedrops or ointment, you may have a terrible taste in your mouth and white specks on the surface of your eye after using the eyedrops or ointment.

Side effects that are potentially life-threatening

Only a small number of persons who take or use ciprofloxacin have major negative effects.

They are less likely to occur while using eyedrops, eye ointment, or eardrops, for example.

These significant side effects can occur in less than one out of every hundred patients. If you get any of the following symptoms, stop taking ciprofloxacin and call your doctor right once.

Muscle weakness, joint discomfort, or swelling in your tendons or joints are all possible symptoms. This is most commonly felt in the ankle or calf, although it can also be felt in the shoulder, arms, or legs. It can begin during the first 2 days of starting ciprofloxacin treatment and can last for several months after ending treatment. It is more frequent in children than in adults.

Pain or odd sensations (such as pins and needles that don't go away, tingling, tickling, numbness, or burning) or weakness in your body, particularly in your legs or arms, are signs of diabetes.

extreme fatigue, feeling frightened or depressed, having trouble sleeping or remembering things, having ringing in your ears (tinnitus), losing your sense of taste, seeing double, or experiencing any other changes in your senses of sight, smell, taste, or hearing are all possible symptoms.

diarrhea (perhaps accompanied by muscular cramps) that contains blood or mucus - if you have severe diarrhea without blood or mucus for more than 4 days, you should see a doctor. a quicker or irregular heartbeat, or heartbeats that become more obvious abruptly (palpitations)

abrupt shortness of breath, especially while sitting down swelling ankles, feet, or stomach convulsions or seizures-like episodes (this side effect can happen if you have epilepsy)

CHAPTER 5

Precautions while using other medications

Some medications have the potential to interfere with the effectiveness of ciprofloxacin. They might also increase your chances of experiencing negative effects.

You must inform your doctor if you are taking any of the following medications prior to taking ciprofloxacin:

If you use antacids for heartburn or indigestion, you should take ciprofloxacin at least 2 hours after you take the tablets. Do not take another antacid for at least 4 hours after you

have taken your ciprofloxacin
methotrexate, a medication used to
treat conditions such as rheumatoid
arthritis phenytoin, a medication used to
treat epilepsy steroids, such as
prednisolone theophylline or
aminophylline for asthma tizanidine, a
medication used to treat muscle
stiffness warfarin, a blood thinner Do
not take another (anticoagulant)

Combining ciprofloxacin with herbal
therapies and dietary supplements is
not recommended.

Ciprofloxacin can be affected by iron
pills (such as ferrous sulphate or ferrous
fumarate), calcium supplements, and
zinc supplements. Allow 2 hours
between each administration of these

supplements and each dose of ciprofloxacin.

There are no documented side effects associated with the use of other vitamins and herbal treatments in conjunction with ciprofloxacin.

CHAPTER 6

WARNING:

Taking ciprofloxacin increases your risk of developing tendinitis (swelling of a fibrous tissue that connects a bone to muscle) or having your tendon ruptured (tearing of a fibrous tissue that connects a bone to a muscle) during your treatment or for up to several months after you finish your treatment. These issues may impact the tendons in your shoulder, your hand, the rear of your ankle, or other regions of your body, among other things. Even while tendinitis or tendon rupture can occur at any age, those over 60 years of age are at the greatest risk for developing the condition. (a disease in which the body attacks its own joints, causing pain, swelling, and loss of function), or if you engage in regular physical activity on a consistent basis. Inform your doctor and pharmacist if you are using oral or injectable steroids, such as dexamethasone, methylprednisolone (Medrol), or prednisone, and if you have any questions or concerns (Rayos). Pain, swelling, soreness, stiffness, or trouble moving a muscle are all signs of tendinitis. Stop taking ciprofloxacin and get medical attention immediately if you suffer any of these symptoms. Take ciprofloxacin immediately and seek emergency medical attention if you suffer any of the following signs of tendon rupture: Injuries to the tendon region can be accompanied by hearing or feeling a snap or pop in the tendon area, bruising in the tendon area following the injury, and difficulty to move or bear weight on the injured area.

Taken in combination with other antibiotics, ciprofloxacin might cause changes in sensation and nerve damage that may persist long after you stop taking the antibiotic. It is possible that this harm will develop shortly after you begin using ciprofloxacin. Inform your physician if you have ever experienced peripheral neuropathy (a type of nerve damage that causes tingling, numbness, and pain in the hands and feet). You should stop taking ciprofloxacin and contact your doctor immediately if you suffer any of the following symptoms: Arms or legs that are numb or tingling, hurting, burning, or have weakness; or a change in your capacity to sense light touch or vibrations; pain; heat or cold; or a change in your ability to feel pain or heat.

Ciprofloxacin may have an adverse effect on your brain or neurological system, resulting in significant side effects. Following the first dose of ciprofloxacin, this is a possibility. As soon as you notice any of these symptoms, call your doctor. If you have seizures or epilepsy, cerebral arteriosclerosis (narrowing of blood arteries in or around the brain that can lead to a ministroke or stroke), stroke, altered brain structure, or renal illness, tell your doctor. You should stop taking ciprofloxacin and contact your doctor immediately if you suffer any of the following symptoms: seizure; tremors; dizziness; lightheadedness; headaches that won't go away (with or without blurred vision); difficulty falling asleep or staying asleep; nightmares; not trusting others or believing that others want to hurt you; hallucinations (seeing things or hearing voices that do not exist); thoughts or actions that lead to harming or killing yourself; feeling restless, anxious, nervous, depressed, confused, or other changes in mood or behavior

It has been reported that taking ciprofloxacin can increase muscular weakness in patients with myasthenia gravis (a nervous system illness that causes muscle weakness), and that it might cause serious difficulties breathing or even death. If you have myasthenia gravis, you should tell your doctor. It is possible that your doctor will advise you not to use ciprofloxacin. You should contact your doctor immediately if you have muscular weakness or trouble breathing while receiving ciprofloxacin therapy if you have myasthenia gravis and your doctor has prescribed this medication.

Inquire with your doctor about the dangers associated with the use of ciprofloxacin.

CHAPTER 7

HOW TO STORE CIPROFLOXACIN

What information should I be aware of about the storage and disposal of this medication?

Keep this medication in the original container it came in, securely closed, and out of the reach of children at all times. Store the tablets and extended-release tablets at room temperature, away from sources of extreme heat and moisture, and away from children (not in the bathroom). Up to 14 days can be spent storing the suspension in the refrigerator or at room temperature, with the lid well closed. Ciprofloxacin suspension should not be frozen. After

14 days, whatever suspension that has remained should be discarded.

NOTE

IMPORTANT DETAILS TO NOTE DOWN

THE END